Journaling to Reclaim the Passion;

A Writing Guide for Nurses

By Kristin Baird, RN, BSN, MHA

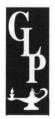 Golden Lamp Press

"Forget all the rules. Forget about being published. Write for yourself and celebrate writing."

-Melinda Haynes

Contents

Introduction

B elieve it or not, you have stories to tell. Even if they are not for anyone else's ears or eyes, your stories can help you to re-connect to your own inner passion for the nursing profession.

Being a nurse means many things to us on many levels. Intellectually, it's the accomplishment of years of study, passing boards and advanced certification, all of which give validation to our intellectual abilities as health professionals. Emotionally, it satisfies a desire to make a contribution for the good of the world through caring and compassion. For some of us this is a spiritual quest to heal others and help them to reach wholeness.

Every nurse has moments when he or she is certain, beyond a doubt, that going into nursing was the "right" choice. Those moments are like cool water from an oasis, rich in their ability to rejuvenate and refresh the spirit. They are the points of passion, that, when put to the test with restricting policies, stifling regulations, staffing shortages and budget cuts, will fade to nothing. Our challenge is to rekindle the passion for caring and let it light the corners of our hospitals, clinics, nursing homes and especially our own lives. It is only through this rejuvenation that we can be our very best for our patients and ourselves.

Many of us can recall the first time we administered an injection, inserted an NG tube or started an IV. We can probably even recount the first code blue, death or birth we witnessed. But how many critical events are lost from our memories, yet held forever by the people whose lives we've touched? Many of us are so adept at caring, compassion and little acts of kindness that it's all in a day's work. We fail to recognize the impact we have on others. While we cannot possibly recall every patient contact with any level of detail, chances are, our patients remember us. Do they remember us for life-saving heroics? Perhaps, but much more likely they remember us for less dramatic feats.

Health care settings are incredible places. While they are a second home to nurses, they are often terrifying places for our patients. Sterile smells, loud, intimidating machines, foreign-sounding terminology spoken by harried, uniformed professionals, painful procedures and dehumanizing gowns are just a few of the amenities we offer our patients. They are vulnerable, frightened and often in pain – both physically and emotionally when arrive in our clinics, hospitals and skilled nursing facilities.

Is it really any wonder that our patients clearly remember the nurse who stayed with them until a family member arrived after an accident? Or held their hand through a long, hard labor? Or brought them a chocolate milk shake to celebrate their progress in physical therapy? Or brought their child a cake when he was hospitalized on his birthday? These acts of kindness are all in a day's work for many nurses, but they are among the hallmarks of our profession.

Nursing is not a spectator sport. As a profession we are there for the births, deaths and all the traumas and illnesses that life deals out in between. In fact, we are so accustomed to being in the middle of it all that many nurses I interviewed had trouble thinking of a time that they felt made a difference. In their minds, it's all in a day's work. The reality is quite the contrary. There are few other professions out there that can claim what we, as nurses, can. In just a half hour's time, we can make a difference in the life of a patient and the lives of that patient's family. We may care for thousands of people in the course of our careers, and after awhile, many of the stories just blend together or are lost. But to the people whose lives we touch, our actions and words are often etched in their memories forever.

Wouldn't it be great if the world could really understand what the nursing profession is all about? It would be so gratifying to have the public see us in reality rather than labeling nurses as the personalities depicted on TV and in the movies. Storytelling is one tool that will help us to accomplish this objective. By telling our stories, nurses will be able to give the world a more realistic view of this profession of ours. Keeping a journal of your own is one way that you can help to contribute to creating a realistic view.

As a consultant, I am often asked to do focus groups for my

healthcare clients. One of my favorite ice breakers is to ask participants to identify their favorite healthcare character from TV or movies. It is rare that any of them mentions a nurse. More often than not they cite a doctor, even when the program they reference has prominent nurse characters. When nurses are mentioned, it is usually for some outrageous character trait rather than for leadership, competency or compassion. I cringe when Margaret "Hot Lips" Houlihan from *M*A*S*H* or Nurse Ratched from ***One Flew Over the Cuckoos Nest*** are mentioned. While Margaret Houlihan is portrayed as a strong nurse-leader, she is also painted as a flirtatious, neurotic sex object. And Nurse Ratched, while strong, is not a nurse I would care to have if my life depended on it.

It's time that nurses tell their own stories. Rather than entrusting our image and purpose to screenplay writers, we can and should take the lead in defining ourselves and letting the world know what we do and what inspires us to do it. The companion book, ***Reclaiming the Passion; Stories That Celebrate the Essence of Nursing*** is a collection of nurses' stories that focus not on life-saving heroics or clinical skills, but on tales of personal passion that reveal the real essence of nursing. But beyond inspiring reading, this book and journal, are intended to be an affirming, interactive process.

As you read through this collection of stories, use this workbook/journal to recall your own stories. Consider forming a Reclaiming the Passion story group at your health care facility. Many nurses struggle with articulating their stories. Sharing your experiences with small peer groups is a good way to become more comfortable with story-telling and through that process to enhance the service culture of your organization.

This journal is a journey back to help you to move forward. When we look back, each of us has a unique opportunity to embrace our past, to forgive mistakes made, to laugh at our naiveté and to gain a psychological lift from seeing the past through our more mature and experienced eyes.

"The journey is the reward."

-*Taoist Saying*

🪔 Preface

Y ou've helped others... now help yourself. Use the tools in this journal to help you look back and understand the choices you have made. Let go of the rules of English and grammar. This isn't a doctoral dissertation to be reviewed and critiqued, but rather personal journaling for your own growth.

Why take this journey? Self-discovery and self-appreciation are two of the main reasons I encourage nurses to write their stories. We are not spectators. We're often right in the middle of the action and yet very few of us see ourselves as the everyday heroes that we are. This exercise isn't striving for a Pulitzer Prize. It's about achieving a better understanding of yourself, your choices, and your personal growth.

Read the book, **Reclaiming the Passion** and use the journal as a series of personal enrichment exercises. The process is designed to leave the nurse/writer with three things: to learn to tell your stories, to cherish your unique contributions and to reflect upon how your work helps to enrich lives – including your own.

This journal contains exercises to help you reclaim your passion for nursing. Following the suggested exercises will help you make the journey back to some of the momentous events in your career that helped to shape the professional you are today. Designed to jog your memory and open your heart, these journal activities will help to get you thinking about your personal relationship with nursing. Enclosed, you will find a CD of beautiful, meditative piano music by Tammie (T.C.) Heintzman, RN. Tammie is a hospice nurse and gifted pianist whose music is often inspired by her patients. (Three of Tammie's stories are included in **Reclaiming the Pasion**.)

I recommend that you find a quiet, comfortable place where you can sit, listen to the CD and write from your heart.

Read the memory joggers at the beginning of each section. Spend a few moments reflecting on the topic and write down your thoughts. I recommend that you refrain from going back over your writing or editing. This is an exercise to help you get your thoughts down on paper. There will be plenty of opportunity later to rewrite if you choose, but for now, focus on simply writing it all down.

If you have never kept a journal before, here are some guidelines that may help you:

- Use the sample questions as a guide, but don't limit yourself. Keep writing even if it means having a separate spiral notebook to catch the overflow.

- Read the companion book, **Reclaiming the Passion; Stories that Celebrate the Essence of Nursing.** Many of the nursing stories included in that book will jog your own memories of similar situations. Use the book as a guide to help you with your personal discovery.

- Take a few moments to reflect before putting the pen to the paper. Be careful not to edit your flow on thoughts; just write them down.

- Write as if you are the only one who will ever read your words. After all, this is your story.

Happy writing!

Kristin Baird

"You don't need to focus on the entire staircase to lift your foot up to the first step."

-Martin Luther King

In the Beginning...

This section will help you to discover some of your earliest ideas about nurses and nursing. Perhaps you had a serious illness that caused you to be hospitalized as a child. Or maybe your only contact with nurses was at the doctor's office for immunizations and well child check ups. Think back to your earliest memories.

- As a child, I thought nurses were...

- Some of the nurses I remember from my childhood were... List them by name or describe their characteristics.

- Can you recall an illness or hospitalization at some point in your youth that made you come in contact with nurses?

- What do you recall? How did you feel about the nurses you encountered?

For many of us, our role in our families helped us to find our strengths and determine our choice of careers.

- Growing up, my role in the family was...

- As a child I felt good about myself when...

- People often praised me for...

- My role in the family may have played a part in my decision to become a nurse by ...

"A journey of a thousand miles begins with a single step."

-Confucius

Classes and Clinicals and Boards, Oh, My!

ost of us have a range of memories from nursing school. Read "School Days" in *Reclaiming the Passion* for some recollections about nursing school.

- I started considering nursing school when...

- Some of my fears about nursing were...

- My greatest struggle in nursing school was...

- My greatest strength in nursing school was..

- How did your parents, family or closest friends react to your decision to attend nursing school? Were they positive and supportive? Did anyone try to discourage you?

- One nursing instructor from my school that stands out in my mind is...

- The best role model I had in school was _____. He/she was outstanding because...

- Describe your classmates in nursing school. Who were your closest friends? What did you do together? Why were they special to you?

- What was your favorite subject?
  What was your least favorite subject?

- What was it like preparing for clinical?

"Unless you try to do something beyond what you have already mastered, you will never grow."

-Ralph Waldo Emerson

It's Often the "Firsts" that Stand Out in Our Minds

C an you recall the first time that you administered an injection? Describe how you felt about giving that first shot.

- What was your first encounter with a dying patient? Think about your reactions and feelings.

- How would you compare your reaction at that time to what you might feel now in a similar situation?

- Describe the first time that you knew you had made a difference for a patient.

- Describe the first time you decided to bend the rules for the benefit of a patient.

- At which organization did you accept your first nursing job?

- What did you learn about yourself in that first job?

_____

_____

_____

_____

_____

_____

_____

_____

_____

"Use what talents you possess: the woods would be very silent if no birds sang except those that sang best."

-Henry Van Dyke

Sharing Your Gifts

For some of us, sharing our gifts is second nature. But for others, there is an invisible boundary that whispers to us to keep a distance and not take chances. Read about how some nurses have shared their gifts in *Reclaiming the Passion*. In the story "Music for the Soul", Tammie Heintzman demonstrates how she shares her gift of music with her hospice patients.

- What gifts do you share with your patients?

- What barriers or inhibitions keep you from sharing more with your patients?

- How do you maintain a balance with boundaries?

"You cannot make yourself feel something you do not feel, but you can make yourself do right in spite of your feelings."

–Pearl S. Buck

🪔 Standing in Judgement

H as there been a time when you have judged a patient only to realize later that you were wrong?

Read the stories, "Just One of Us" and "Holding Up a Mirror" in *Reclaiming the Passion*. Think about the experiences shared by Lisa Harris and Kathy Hageseth in their stories, then reflect on a time when you may have passed judgment on a patient. Write about your feelings.

- Did someone else point out your judgmental attitude? If so, how did you feel about the encounter and what did you learn?

- How have these lessons helped you in your practice?

- If you work with someone who is judgmental of patients, what lesson or information would you like to share with him or her?

- How could you use your own experience to help them grow?

_____

_____

_____

_____

_____

_____

_____

_____

_____

_____

"We must embrace pain and burn it as fuel for our journey."

-Kenji Miyazawa

Swallow Hard and Keep Going

R ead "No Time for Tears" in **Reclaiming the Passion** and reflect. Have you had times when you felt like shutting down after an emotional encounter with a patient, but had to keep going? How did you cope?

- Write about a time when you questioned the value of your work. What seems to trigger your "down times" in nursing?

- How do you rise above these challenges to reclaim your passion for nursing?

_____

_____

_____

_____

_____

_____

_____

_____

_____

_____

_____

_____

_____

_____

_____

"Helping people in need is a good and essential part of my life, a kind of destiny."

-Princess Diana

Listening

There are so many times when we need to move past a patient's words to discover the essence of their needs. Read "Listening with Heart" in *Reclaiming the Passion* and reflect on the following:

- Think back on a time when you were truly an excellent listener for a patient. Consider how you saw beyond the words or tangible information to understand, then reach the patient.

- Is there someone you know that is an incredible listener? What behaviors do they demonstrate that make you feel valued and heard?

- How can you apply those skills in your own actions?

_____

_____

_____

_____

_____

_____

_____

_____

_____

_____

_____

_____

_____

_____

"Presence is more than just being there."

-*Malcolm S. Forbes*

The Power of Your Presence

We often place such value in doing that we forget the power of just being there for someone else. Read "A Very Special Delivery" and "Thank you, Howard" in *Reclaiming the Passion*. Consider your personal experiences involving patient grief.

- Describe a time when you demonstrated that you were truly there for a patient and family. How did you feel? What was the patient's response? What could you have done differently?

- Recall a time when your presence was all that was needed to comfort someone else. What did you learn from the experience?

- Think of a time when all *you* needed was someone to stay beside you. How did you feel about truly needing someone else? How did that person's presence make you feel?

_____

_____

_____

_____

_____

_____

_____

_____

_____

_____

_____

"True feeling justifies whatever it may cost."

-May Sarton

🪔 Gut Feelings

H ave you ever had a gut feeling about a patient's condition that defied concrete evidence and yet proved to be your best guide? Read "The Feeling" in *Reclaiming the Passion*.

- How much value do you place in your personal intuition about your patients?

- Describe a time when intuition helped guide you toward the best actions for your patients.

_____

_____

_____

_____

_____

_____

_____

_____

_____

_____

_____

_____

_____

_____

_____

_____

"To teach is to learn twice."

–Joseph Joubert

Teachers and Students

Teaching is a natural part of nursing. Whether it is teaching patients how to prevent illness or how to optimize their health in spite of a chronic disease, nurses continually impart information that improves others' quality of life. But through teaching others, we often become the student, taking away rich experiences. Read "Making the Dean's List" in *Reclaiming the Passion*.

- Reflect on times when you taught others. It could be as specific as teaching a technical skill or as broad as being a preceptor for a newly hired nurse. What did you learn about yourself when you became the teacher? Did teaching help you enhance your own skills? Did it help boost your enthusiasm?

- How confident are you in teaching others?

- What steps can you take to enhance your teaching abilities? Think of an example where teaching someone else helped you to see a situation through new eyes. What (if anything) did the experience change for you?

"To measure the man, measure his heart."

-Malcolm Stevenson Forbes

🪔 Universal Language

A touch, a smile, a well-timed hug are just a few of the non-verbal means we use to communicate compassion, understanding and empathy. Read "The Power of Touch", "A Universal Language" and "Reaching Out from the Dark" in *Reclaiming the Passion*.

- Describe a time when touch was the only comfort measure you had to offer. Consider how the patient reacted. Recall how you felt about their reaction.

- How comfortable are you with touch? If you are often reluctant to reach out and touch someone, what is holding you back?

- Have you ever been the patient? Describe a situation when you felt particularly vulnerable and needed to rely on others to care for you. What did you learn about touch and other forms of nonverbal communication from that experience?

- Think of some examples of times when no words would suffice in comforting a patient. What did you do? How did you feel? What reaction did you get from the patient?

"*Remember, people will judge you by your actions, not your intentions. You may have a heart of gold – but so does a hard-boiled egg.*"

–Anonymous

Between a Rock and a Hard Place

There are times when nurses are caught between a patient's desires and accepted protocol, doctors orders or even a Power of Attorney's wishes. Read "The Feeling" and "Patient Advocacy" in *Reclaiming the Passion*.

- When have you felt caught between a patient's desires and other demands? How did you feel about being in that position? In hind sight, what did you learn? Would you have done anything differently than what you did at the time?

- Are there recurrent dilemmas in your practice that make you feel torn? Describe them.

_____

_____

_____

_____

_____

_____

_____

_____

_____

_____

_____

_____

_____

_____

"There is no place for dogma in science. The scientist is free, and must be free to ask any question, to doubt any assertion, to seek for any evidence, to correct any errors."

-J. Robert Oppenheimer

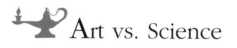

Art vs. Science

How do you practice the art of nursing? How do you balance the art with the science? In **Reclaiming the Passion**, read "The Art of Nursing", based on an interview with Karen Lee Fontaine.

The science part of nursing is pretty straightforward. What are some of the challenges you face in the scientific part of nursing?

Creativity is a great asset in nursing. There are often times when nurses must rely on their own resourcefulness to tackle problems. We build confidence when we exercise critical thinking and find solutions to problems through innovation. Read "Olympic Moments" in **Reclaiming the Passion**. Think of times when you came up with unique solutions to problems.

- What do you like about science? What do you dislike?

- How do you define the "art" of nursing?

- What struggles, if any, do you have in balancing the art of nursing with the science?

- Do you find yourself gravitating more toward the art or the science in nursing? Does one have greater intrigue and rewards over the other? Why?

_____

_____

_____

_____

_____

_____

"If I can put one touch of rosy sunset into the life of any man or woman, I shall feel that I have worked with God."

–Gilbert K. Chesterton

Spiritually Speaking

Many nurses talk about nursing as a way to incorporate their spiritual beliefs with their careers. Reflect on your own personal, spiritual beliefs and how you bridge these with your nursing practice. Read "A personal Ministry" and "A Great Return on Investment" in *Reclaiming the Passion* for two nurses' perspectives on blending work and beliefs.

- How comfortable are you with talking to patients about their spiritual beliefs?

- How do you approach patients whose spiritual beliefs are in direct contrast to your own?

- What are your beliefs about spirituality and healing? Do these beliefs help you in doing your work? If so, how?

"Experience is not what happens to you; it's what you do with what happens to you."

-*Aldous Huxley*

What We Learn Through the Pain

Read "The Final Call" and "Thank You, Howard" in *Reclaiming the Passion*. Reflect on times when you were there for a dying patient. How did you handle your own personal grief? What did you learn about yourself and your own beliefs about death by helping someone else at the end of his or her life?

Read "Honoring What is Sacred" in *Reclaiming the Passion*. Reflect on your own experiences in dealing with cultural or religious traditions different from your own. Have you had experiences where the patient's beliefs required that you bend the hospital, agency or clinic rules in order to accommodate their needs? What was the situation? How did you handle it? What would you do differently today?

_____

_____

_____

_____

_____

_____

_____

_____

_____

_____

_____

_____

_____

_____

_____

"Rules are not necessarily sacred, principles are."

-Franklin D. Roosevelt

Breaking the Rules

H ave you ever broken the rules to do what you felt was best for a patient? Read "Bending the Rules" and "Thank You Howard" in *Reclaiming the Passion*. Think back on times when you have chosen to break the rules in the patients' best interest.

• How do you maintain the balance between being the patient advocate and following rules that may not be in your patient's best interest?

• When do you feel it is worth it to break the rules?

_____

_____

_____

_____

_____

_____

_____

_____

_____

_____

_____

_____

_____

_____

_____

_____

"Action expresses priorities."

-Mohandas Gandhi

Boundaries

M any nurses struggle with professional boundaries.

• What messages did you receive about boundaries during nursing school?

• How do you define traditional and professional boundaries?

• How do these definitions fit with your personal views?

• When do we reach out to our patients and families beyond the conventional, clinical interactions? Describe a time when you were glad that you stretched beyond the traditional boundaries.

• Describe a time when you didn't stretch beyond the boundaries only to later regret your decision to hold back.

• If you were training new nurses, what would you like to tell them about boundaries?

_____

_____

_____

_____

_____

_____

_____

_____

_____

"The key is not to prioritize what's on your schedule, but to schedule your priorities."

-Stephen R. Covey

Setting Priorities

There is no shortage of demands for your time every day. But sometimes we catch ourselves placing tasks above human contact. Refer to "Efficiency Isn't Enough" and "A Change in Priorities" in *Reclaiming the Passion*.

Reflect on situations you have experienced where a patient has helped you shift your focus from tasks to more human interaction.

- Write about messages you may have received as a child about productivity vs. 'down time'. Which carried a greater value in your home life – productivity or human relationships? How has this carried over into your nursing practice?

- Have you changed your views about tasks vs. interaction during your career? What have been the most valuable lessons?

"Humor prevents one from becoming a tragic figure even though he or she is involved in tragic events."

-E.T. Eberhart

Laughter is Good Medicine

It is inevitable that you will have funny moments in your line of work. Read "Here's Looking at You" and "Who's Smiling Now" in *Reclaiming the Passion*. Think of times when you have had a good laugh about something at work.

• How do you use humor in your work?

_____

_____

_____

_____

_____

_____

_____

_____

_____

_____

_____

_____

_____

_____

_____

_____

_____

_____

_____

_____

_____

"What is the good of experience if you do not reflect?"

-Frederick the Great

Knowing Yourself

I n order to be happy and fulfilled, each of us must spend time reflecting on what is most important to us. Use the following questions to help gain insight into your needs and values.

- To me the perfect day looks like this...

- When I die, I want to be remembered for...

- The three most important roles that I play in my life are ____, _____ and _____

  - I keep them in balance by...

- I know when I'm in balance physically, emotionally and spiritually when...

- I know I am getting out of balance when...

- I feel most fulfilled when....

_____

_____

_____

_____

_____

_____

_____

_____

_____

"Just as your car runs more smoothly and requires less energy to go faster and farther when the wheels are in perfect alignment, you perform better when your thoughts, feelings, emotions, goals and values are in balance."

–Brian Tracy

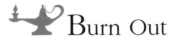Burn Out

Almost everyone has high and low points in the course of his or her career. List your previous jobs and identify what you liked and didn't like about each position. Reflect on your personal needs and how they were or were not met in each situation.

- Have you ever felt truly burned out? Describe the situation. What did you do to get past it?

- How do you seek new challenges?

- Do you get bored with your work easily?

- What do you do to re-energize yourself when you are feeling burned out?

- How do you take care of yourself?

_____

_____

_____

_____

_____

_____

_____

_____

_____

_____

"Enthusiasm is contagious. Be a carrier."

-Susan Rabin

Part of the Solution

When I hear people complaining without considering possible solutions, I ask them if they want to be part of the problem or part of the solution. Complaints without solutions only serve to perpetuate the problem. As nurses, we need to be prepared to speak positively about the work that we do. In doing so, we will be helping to shed a more positive light on the profession.

• Make a list of all of the things you enjoy about nursing.

• How has nursing helped you to grow?

• Has being a nurse helped you to gain confidence? Interact better with others? Expand your horizons?

Consider the opportunities you might have to speak with others about the positive aspects of nursing. Make a habit of speaking positively about your work and about the importance of nurses. Remember that enthusiasm (as well as negativity) is contagious.

• What would you tell young children about what it is like to be a nurse?

• What would you tell teens?

• What would you tell other adults?

_____

_____

_____

_____

_____

"*Try to make at least one person happy every day. If you cannot do a kind deed, speak a kind word. If you cannot speak a kind word, think a kind thought. Count up, if you can, the treasure of happiness that you would dispense in a week, in a year, in a lifetime!*"

–Lawrence G. Lovasik

I Know I Made A Difference Today

This is probably one of the most important sections of your journal. Use this section of the journal to record the small triumphs that help you to remember that you have made a difference in the life of a patient or a patient's family. Of course, for confidentiality reasons, it is important not to mention patients by name even in your private journal.

Read "Maybe Today I Made a Difference" and Just Being There With a Smile" in *Reclaiming the Passion* to remind yourself that it's often the little things that really matter to patients.

Refer back to this list whenever you need to rejuvenate and to re-connect with your passion for nursing. This activity can help you to stay fresh, creative and energized in your work.

_____

_____

_____

_____

_____

_____

_____

_____

_____

_____

_____

_____

"Live your life from your heart. Share from your heart. And your story will touch and heal people's souls."

–Melody Beattie

About the Author

Kristin Baird has over twenty-five years of experience in health care. Baird earned a BSN from the University of Wisconsin-Madison, and has clinical experience ranging from public health to critical care. She earned a Masters of Science in Health Services Administration from Cardinal Stritch College in Milwaukee.

Baird began consulting in 1991, specializing in health care marketing, communications and customer service. She has received more than twenty regional and national awards for health care writing, advertising, marketing and public relations.

Baird is the author of *Customer Service in Healthcare; A Grassroots Approach to Creating a Culture of Service Excellence* (2000. American Hospital Association Publishing and Jossey-Bass).

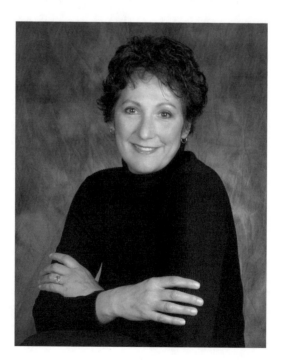

About the Companion Book

merica's nurses are without question among the most highly skilled of all medical practitioners. Yet at some point every nurse discovers that skills are not enough. Through dozens of interviews with nurses from around the United States, Baird helps readers to rediscover passion as an essential trait of their profession. Written for nurses, about nurses and by a nurse, *Reclaiming the Passion; Stories that Celebrate the Essence of Nursing* taps into the most humanizing elements of nursing to offer motivation at a time when the profession cries out for a spark of inspiration.

Baird's stories are not about lifesaving heroics. Rather they are about individual epiphanies, moments of truth that emerge between patients and their care givers, leaving both better for having shared even a brief time together.

To order your copy of *Reclaiming the Pasison*, please log onto
www.reclaimingthepassion.com
or see the attached order form on page 221 of this journal.

🕯Popular Presentations by Kristin Baird

Reclaiming the Passion — Celebrating the Essence of Nursing

This motivational presentation developed specifically for nurses will have you laughing, crying and re-affirming your commitment to the nursing profession. Baird uses storytelling about everyday people and the lessons they learned in trenches of the nursing profession. She reminds nurses to cherish their unique contributions and to reflect upon how their work shapes lives — including their own. This presentation is ideal for health care organizations that want to salute their nurses and celebrate the profession, whether it's through Nurses Day celebrations (May) or ongoing recruitment and retention initiatives.

Customer Service in Healthcare — Creating a Culture of Service Excellence

Based on personal experience, Baird shares steps to creating a service-centered culture in health care settings. Her witty, yet practical approach leaves her audiences spinning with take-home ideas for implementation. Baird takes her audiences through the common pitfalls of customer service programs and leaves them with a list of practical tips and feeling inspired to facilitate change. This presentation is appropriate for anyone working in health care. It is a popular program for helping employees at all levels of the organization to see their vital role in customer service.

Quality Through the Eyes of the Beholder — the Customer Service Link

Baird takes her audiences out of the traditional definitions of quality and helps them to see quality through the eyes of their customers. Using storytelling, skillfully combined with data, Baird demonstrates the link between service and a healthy bottom line. Baird encourages her audiences to embrace customer service at all levels of their organization. This presentation is appropriate for health care managers and senior leadership but can be tailored to other service industries as well. Components are used in a keynote or extended into a full day workshop. The full day workshop contains exercises to help participants hone the skills necessary in leading a service initiative within their own organization.

Kris Baird is an amazing speaker. She combines professional credibility, practical knowledge, humor, personal insight and effective speaking style into a very effective presentation. Ms Baird was the highlight of my Public Relations conference, receiving an "excellent" rating from every attendee.

– Kevin Stranberg
    Conference Planner, WHPRMS

Kris' interactive sessions were very well received and she sparked renewed enthusiasm for customer service.

– Tolly Arthur
    Director of Marketing
    Medical Associates Health Centers

I was so impressed with her presentation that I knew I wanted her to speak at our Iowa conference.

– Danice Larson, RN CPHQ
    President-Elect IAHQ

For more information about keynote presentations, speeches, workshops
and consulting by Kristin Baird, please call
Baird Consulting, Inc. at (920) 563-4684 or log onto
www.baird-consulting.com.

I have a passion for nursing!

Please contact me with more information on:

___ starting a storytelling group within my organization.
___ placing a bulk order of books/journals for my
       organization's nurses. Discounts are available.
___ inviting Kristin Baird to speak at my organization.
___ placing me on your mailing list for information on
       upcoming editions of *Reclaiming the Passion.*

* If you have checked any of the above, please provide the following
information for follow-up:

Name ———————————————————————————

Organization ————————————————————————

Phone ————————— E-mail ———————————————

Address ——————————————————————————

City————————————— State ———— Zip ——————————

Please submit this form by fax: (920) 563-3777 or by mail:
Golden Lamp Press, P.O. Box 622 Fort Atkinson, WI 53538

To place an order for *Reclaiming the Passion* or *Journaling to Reclaim the Passion,*
or to share your story, please long onto **www.reclaimingthepassion.com**. For
general information on Kristin Baird and her work, please log onto:
www.baird-consulting.com.

Thanks for helping nurses to tell the stories of their great work!

Order Form

Item Description	Quantity	Cost per unit	Subtotal
Reclaiming the Passion – Book (1 unit)		x $15.95	
Journaling to Reclaim the Passion – Journal and CD (1 unit)		x $22.95	
Gift Set – Book, journal & music CD (1 unit)		x $35.00	
Subtotal			
Shipping & Handling		x $5.75/unit	
Total			

Method of Payment

☐ Check/ Money Order enclosed   ☐ Charge to:
       ❏ Master Card
       ❏ Visa

Card # _____

Expiration Date _____

_____
Signature of Card Holder

Order online with credit card at www.reclaimingthepassion.com.

Make checks payable to:
Golden Lamp Press, LLC

Mail orders to:
Golden Lamp Press
PO Box #622
Fort Atkinson, WI 53538

Ship to:

Name _____
Organization _____
Phone _____ E-mail _____
Address _____
City _____ State _____ Zip _____

Tell Us What You Think!

Dear friends,

This journal came about through years of listening. Your feedback is valuable to future editions of *Reclaiming the Passion*. Please send us your comments and suggestions by copying and completing the brief questionnaire on the following pages. You may fax your completed form to: (920) 563-3777 or complete the survey online by logging onto:

www.reclaimingthepassion.com.

Thank you in advance for your support.

Kindest Regards,

Kristin Baird

Reader Feedback

To:
Kristin Baird, RN
Golden Lamp Press
P.O. Box 622   Fax: (920) 563-3777
Fort Atkinson, WI 53538   Email: info@reclaimingthepassion.com

From:

Name _____

Address _____

City _____ State _____ Zip_____

Phone _____ fax_____

e-mail _____

I became aware of *Journaling to Reclaim the Passion* through:

❏ a friend's recommendation
❏ a web search
❏ a magazine/journal article
❏ the book *Reclaiming the Passion*
❏ other (please explain)

My favorite section was _____

One thing I learned about myself through journaling was

_____

_____

I have a copy of *Reclaiming the Passion*

❏ Yes   ❏ No
    If yes:
    • How would you rate the book? (1 = not at all useful, 5 = very useful)

1   2   3   4   5

On a scale of 1-5 please rate *Journaling to Reclaim the Passion;
A Writing Guide for Nurses*:

	Very Poor	Poor	Average	Good	Excellent
Writing cues for personal reflection	1	2	3	4	5
Inspirational quotes	1	2	3	4	5
Value received for the cost of the journal	1	2	3	4	5

How likely are you to:

	Not at all likely	Somewhat likely	Not sure	Somewhat likely	Very likely
Recommend this journal to a friend	1	2	3	4	5
Purchase future editions of *Reclaiming the Passion*	1	2	3	4	5
Share one of your own stories	1	2	3	4	5

How could we have made the book better?

What would you like to see changed for future editions?